CONTENTS

INTRODUCTION

If you were asked to list the ideal qualifications for writing a book on cerebral palsy for parents, you would probably name at least two. First, the author should be intimately acquainted with many different people with this disorder, since it is so varied that a limited contact would never be adequate. Second, he should be equally well acquainted with the agencies serving the cerebral palsied, the strengths and the pitfalls of these agencies, and how "rehabilitation" can easily lead to debilitation.

The author of this book, Gil Joel, not only meets these qualifications but fulfills them on the highest level. The most essential of his qualifications is the fact that he can view cerebral palsy from a special vantage point, and it is therefore important for me to introduce the author and not merely the book. Gil has *lived* cerebral palsy and experienced its manifold problems because he is afflicted with a severe form of this disorder. He has learned, over the years, how to accept this condition without surrendering to it, how to achieve independence when others expected or even invited dependence, how to maintain a positive self-image in the face of a negative body image, and how to develop and give expression to abilities which, with less effort on his part and less encouragement from his family, could have remained latent and unrecognized to this day.

These personal experiences have reached their culmination in this down-to-earth, mind-expanding guide for all parents of children with cerebral palsy. It is ideally suited not only to individual use, but as a stimulus for an exchange of ideas with other parents, since it deals with every major question and problem that is bound to arise in the family: the importance of early and exact diagnosis, the different types of treatment and rehabilitation, the relation between independence and self-sufficiency, the pitfalls of sheltered workshops and rehab centers, practical pointers for "outsmarting" this handicap, home vs. residential care, and the more personal but always vital questions of affection, sex, and marriage. Also, the use of cerebral palsy as a focal point is a wise choice because in this disorder the effects of virtually every other disability are represented.

For this reason the book can be of immense indirect benefit to parents if it is assigned, as it should be, as basic reading for students in special education and rehabilitation courses—and, indeed, if it is read by all other students in high school and college who become interested in the problems of the disabled. For the ideas on which this book is based can be applied not only to the cerebral palsied but to practically all of the thirty million or more in our population who must face a disability of one kind or another. As Gil Joel trenchantly points out, every person with a special problem must be accepted as an integral member of society, with the same essential hopes and aspirations, the same general kinds of challenges, and the same need as everyone else to develop his capacities to the utmost and enjoy life to the fullest possible degree.

Gil Joel's book, with its positive, constructive approach, goes a long way toward showing how this can be done.

Robert M. Goldenson, Ph.D.
author of *The Encyclopedia of
Human Behavior* and *Psychology, Psychiatry,
and Mental Health*

PREFACE

While it would boost my ego to think that this book is the result of my many years of counseling the parents of cerebral palsied children and of advising CP adults, I must admit that it is actually the result of a childhood frustrated by inability to get through to my mother and father what it is really like to be a CP.

I have spent much of my professional writing career trying again and again to address myself to my own parents. I am not unaware of the problems faced by parents of CP children, and, to a great extent, this book is dedicated to making the life of the parent easier.

At the same time, however, I owe it to myself and my fellow CPs to get across to you what we feel.

For example, it is not easy for one who is to some extent dependent on other people for his basic needs to feel comfortable with them—let alone equal.

Satirist Mort Sahl has a passion for nailing loose-talking people to the wall by insisting: "Define your terms!" Old Mort would have a field day with relatives and friends of the handicapped. There are countless terms flung around every day which cry out to be defined. Among these are "happy, useful citizen," "self-sufficient," "independent," "an inspiration to others."

We CPs hear these terms constantly. We grew up with them. But their meaning is lost to us because they no longer have meaning. Handicapped or not, the "self-made man" is as extinct as the Brontosaurus. The "happy, useful citizen" is neither happy nor useful unless he knows that both his happiness and his usefulness are gifts from people and must be passed on to other people.

No one, not even the artist or the farmer, is either "self-sufficient" or "independent." The strength of our society comes, oddly enough, from man's dependence upon his fellow man.

Why should this not be true for the cerebral palsied?

Actually, the meaningless platitudes about independence, usefulness, and self-sufficiency regarding the handicapped are simply desperate attempts to reverse the thinking of the so-called normal who through the centuries have regarded the handicapped as helpless and useless. Perhaps the theory is that all wrongs committed against the handicapped can be made right just by changing "They can do nothing" to "They can do anything."

This attitude in itself is bad enough, but matters are made worse when the "normal" world implies that the handicapped "can do anything *by themselves*." If a person with no physical limitations needs help from those around him, how can the handicapped be expected to achieve independence?

At this point, your response might be: "But everybody knows that when we talk about independence we are aware that all of us need some help."

Well, this may or may not be true. The only reason I raise the issue at all is that the nonhandicapped seem to think otherwise about the disabled. How many people do you know who got a good job without a word in the right place from the right person? Yet we expect the handicapped person to do the Horatio Alger bit and get his own job or build his own business. How many married couples do you know who were not helped to the altar by friends? Yet we expect the handicapped to live alone in the unnatural state of singleness. How many doors would we allow to slam in the face of a normal stranger? Yet we hesitate to help a handicapped person because "he might resent it." How many total strangers would we eject from our cocktail parties? Yet we do not think to invite our handicapped friends. "They wouldn't fit in," we say. "They're quite independent, you know. Much more comfortable by themselves."

And now let us take a closer look at the one who is "an inspiration to others." Who is he? To whom is he an inspiration?

He is, of course, that mythological "self-made man." Whether or not he had help in achieving whatever status he had doesn't really matter. He is an inspiration to us by virtue of the fact that he never asked *us* to help him. For if we had been involved in his success, he would be "a living example of what can be accomplished when people care."

Thus I submit that there is in truth no such thing as self-help—for the handicapped or anyone else.

God helps those who help themselves by helping us to help each other.

A NOTE TO THE READER

Before you proceed into this book, I think I should clarify two points. First, the use of the term "CP child" rather than "child who has cerebral palsy" may appear to contradict a statement made early in the book that you should not think of your child as a handicapped child but rather as a child who happens to have a handicap. "CP child" is, I feel, a correct term because it stands for "cerebral pals*ied*" child, that is, a child who has cerebral palsy. Also, it happens to be easier to read.

In my discussion of sheltered workshops, I deliberately avoided specifying which handicapped people now benefit from this service. I did so because I consider it irrelevant that at this particular time no better way has been found to make certain people feel important to themselves and their world. This is a transitory condition which will, I am sure, rectify itself when our society realizes that sheltered workshops operate on the Marxist principle that a man is valued by his rate of production. This is not the measure of a man. Effort, integrity, humanness, dedication, and love are far better measures than production. I pass lightly over sheltered workshops in this book in the hope that they will go away.

1

"What's Wrong with My Baby?"

OK. So you played the percentages and you lost. Your child was born with cerebral palsy. Well, the truth is that his chances of being born normal weren't as great as you think. After all, one of us CPs is born every fifty-three minutes in the United States alone.

This little statistic doesn't make you feel any better. Even if my parents had known, it wouldn't have comforted them. Nothing would have, except perhaps the chance to peer thirty years into the future.

Millions of words have already been written about the all-consuming guilt shared by parents of CP children. Now it may be perfectly true that a good number of parents actually feel they're being punished for some real or imagined sin of their past, but my experience suggests that this guilt feeling is not as common as the experts claim. I've talked with quite a few parents about this. Suppose I start with my own.

Like many CPs, I looked normal at birth. An early case of jaundice transformed my appearance. "When they brought you to me all covered up in a blanket," my mother tells me, "and I opened the blanket and saw a yellow, screaming, trembling version of the happy and healthy baby they had shown me the day before, I was really more angry than afraid. My first thought wasn't: 'What's wrong with my baby?' It was: 'What have they done to my baby?' The birth of a child, any child, is a miracle. How could your father and I ever think of a miracle as punishment?"

My mother insists that even if she hadn't felt that the hospital was to blame for my condition she and my father would never have blamed themselves. I know she is sincere because she candidly admits: "Of course, if you had been my first child, I might have wondered if it would be safe for me to have another. But, even so, I still don't think I'd have felt guilty about anything."

My father's answer is more simple and direct: "Guilty? I never did anything to make myself feel guilty!"

It is interesting to me that parents of CPs born prior to 1945 seem more to share my parents' view than do more recent parents, and I think I know why. In the days of the depression, adversity was commonplace. The appearance of a handicapped child on the scene was just one more lump in the oatmeal. Also, people weren't nearly as psychology oriented as they are today. They were less likely to ask themselves why things happened to them. I have no idea whether this was good or bad. I only know it's true.

But why do I choose 1945 as the dividing line? I do so because this was the year that saw the real birth of rehabilitation centers. From then on the parent was no longer alone with his "problem"—if indeed he thought of it

2

as such. Meeting other parents was (and is) often a tremendous help, and on this I'll elaborate later. But fear has a way of spreading, and one fearful, guilt-ridden parent can infect an entire waiting room.

I brought up this guilt question early in order to get it out of the way, for it really is irrelevant. Guilty or not, "sinful" or not, you *are* the parent of a child who may well remain as helpless as an infant long after his infancy. What are you going to do about it? Sooner or later you will have to decide whether you will keep your child at home or place him in an institution. This is a very big question which we'll talk about in Chapter 2. Maybe I'm expounding the obvious, but before you tackle that question you'll have to find out just how handicapped your child is likely to be.

And finding out may not be easy. Even in this day of medical enlightenment, there are scores of family physicians who cannot or will not tell a parent that his child has cerebral palsy. Ridiculous as it seems, there are doctors still unable to recognize cerebral palsy when they see it. Of course, this does happen more often when the child is very young, but it can occur even later. The saddest instance is when a doctor knows the child has cerebral palsy and decides not to tell the parents.

Why will a doctor choose to play God with a family's entire future?

There are several reasons. First, in the back of his mind is the chance that he could be wrong, and if he is, he doesn't want to deliver needlessly a life sentence of hardship, hopelessness, and heartbreak. Second, if he is sure of his diagnosis he figures there is lots of time for the child to begin therapy which might or might not do any good.

3

Meanwhile, he reasons, let the tot be happy in his short-lived freedom and let the parents hope their baby will "outgrow it." Third, he may feel that the immediate family situation is not ripe for such catastrophic news. Maybe in six months or so . . . .

While this problem of diagnosis doesn't affect you now, chances are it is not unfamiliar to you. If you got a straight and true answer from the first or even the fifth doctor you consulted, count yourself lucky. And things were much worse more than forty years ago when I was a baby.

My "baby book" reads like a chronicle of heartbreak. My mother's pitifully brief insertions in the "Physical Progress" column say more about the gnawing hopelessness which had invaded our little family than I could ever convey. She kept these monthly records only until my first birthday.

Yet hopeless as the picture appeared, my mother was still convinced that one day I would "amount to something."

But suppose she had been wrong? She could have been, you know. A few more damaged brain cells would have transformed her intuition into a pipe dream. Or I could have been unlucky enough to be the right person in the wrong place: no big brother to goad me into talking; no friend to play with me like I was "just another kid"; no home teacher to open the world of books to me; no editor willing to take a chance on a novice writer; no girl to see in Gil Joel the man I would never have become without her.

And if my mother had been wrong—if I had been incapable of progress and she had kept me home anyway—consider the injustice to my father, to my brother and sister, to herself! Because your child is your child he is special. But no human being has the right to be so special that he destroys another person. Bear this in mind while you read the next chapter.

4

2

"Should We Put Him Away?"

Think about what I've just said: No one is so special that he has the right to destroy another. I'm not going off on a theological tangent, but this must be the heart of the issue when and if you have to think of placing your handicapped child in an institution, or, as relatives and friends neatly call it, "putting him away."

This is what hurts the most, of course. How can you "put away" a living part of yourself? Outsiders seem to write it off so matter-of-factly. They act as if there were no more to it than junking a damaged car.

But there is more to it. Your child is *your child*. And for this reason alone he is special. Now, however, we approach dangerous territory. Every instinct tells you that the more dependent your child is upon you, the more special he becomes. It isn't, as some will say, that you enjoy being a martyr. It's just that the more time you invest each day in caring for your child, the greater is his hold upon your heart. Face it now before it happens, while you can still be at all objective.

Let us not get into a discussion about how badly disabled your child is. I have no way of seeing for myself, and if I did, I'd be eminently unqualified to make a judgment on a medical matter—although I can point out that if, like many CPs, your child is also epileptic, the extent of his epilepsy should be taken into account in deciding whether to place him in an institution. In general, I would say that if caring for your child takes up over 25 percent more of your time than caring for any other child, you must consider his future in the household.

These remarks are particularly addressed to you, the mother, for in most cases you spend more time than your husband caring for the child. In the end it is you who can best decide whether your child remains at home or goes to an institution. You must feed, dress, and bathe him. Only you (until doctors and therapists enter the picture) know exactly how much care he needs. Because of all the time you spend together, probably you alone can really communicate with him and, if you let yourself, can most accurately assess his intelligence.

The decision which must be yours is sticky enough when the child is so badly disabled and so severely retarded that you know for sure he wouldn't be aware of his surroundings. Who is to tell you that this child is not worth loving? But if you are capable of weighing all the facts, you will bring yourself to realize that the best way to love him is to lift from him the means of destroying those around him. All you can do for this child can be done just as well in a good institution without sacrificing the happiness of your husband and other children. And if you have no other children, think of the crime it would be to decide to give all your love to this child, who will always consume more of it and digest none of it!

But what about the "question mark" child: the one in whom no one can tell what is hidden behind that contorted, drooling face? Will he always be so helpless? Is there a possibility that his mind is so remarkable that it will one day break through its physical prison and literally outsmart his handicap? It takes a very unusual parent indeed to separate the hopeless case from the child with potential, and to admit when she has made a mistake in judgment. This whole touchy business is still too much a matter of maternal intuition for my liking. Had I been born in 1974 instead of 1928, my mother would have gotten no more help than she did decades ago in finding out my mental capacity. Testing techniques for children who can't communicate either verbally or with hand signals are still in the dark ages.

Here in a nutshell is the parents' dilemma: "If it is true that no person is so special that he has the right to destroy another, and if it is also true that our child might, with the right amount of love and encouragement, develop into someone who loves and is loved by the world around him, are *we* so special that we have the right to destroy him?"

This must be immediately followed by the question: "Would sending the child to an institution really destroy him?"

Unfortunately, there's no pat answer. As far as I was concerned, I doubt that there's an institution in the world that could have given me what my family gave. It wasn't a very stable or materially secure household, but it was mine, and because it was mine it made me feel that even if I couldn't talk or do a thing for myself, I was *somebody!*

On the other hand, I know one young adult who is eternally grateful to her parents for sending her to a training school: "The training I got," she says, "taught me to do more for myself, but that part of it is minor. The important thing I learned was never to allow myself to be so dependent on others for my care that I should ever be sent away again. I feel that my determination to stay in the community has made me work harder to improve myself than all the lectures my parents, doctors, and therapists could have given." This young woman is now happily married.

The decision is yours, but don't try to make it by yourself. Remember that your husband has a stake in this too. Talk it out together from every angle, and as you talk you will find the areas you both must investigate before any decision is reached.

What do the doctors say? Do they feel that as an in-patient at a rehabilitation hospital your child will progress more quickly and completely than he would attending a rehab center two or three days a week? If this is their honest opinion and they are not simply trying to give you an easy out, your duty is clear. Your child may feel rejected at first, but advance and repeated assurances that you are not "putting him away" and regular visits from you will reduce the sting of institutional life. As long as he can still identify with his family, he will know that he *has* connections with the outside world, and he'll be happy.

At this point, I think it's important to spell out the different types of placement that are open to you. Here the three factors involved are your financial circumstances, the age and physical and mental condition of your child, and the resources available in your community. Basically, your choices are: in-patient services at a private, voluntary, or state rehabilitation center (one that prepares the child for life in the community); enrollment in a private, voluntary, or state training school where emphasis is on developmental training (training that is not designed to help the child out of the institution) and activities of daily living rather than on rehabilitation; and custodial care in a private or state institution.

Realize, first of all, that while it is generally true that in each instance private is superior to voluntary and voluntary is superior to state, this is not always true. In New York state, for example, I've seen state-sponsored rehab centers that far surpass centers which are either privately owned or supported by voluntary contributions. By the same token, countless centers sponsored by United Cerebral Palsy and other voluntary agencies are far superior to the most highly rated private institutions.

How do you know which type of residence is right for your child? Well, let's assume for the moment that you have definitely come to the conclusion that your child is not really benefiting from his life at home. The hang-ups are gone, the decision is made, and you are free to find exactly the right place for your child. Great! But forget it!

The hard truth is that the "perfect place" simply does not exist. There *is* no place like home. No place will always give your child the foods he likes best, be at his beck and call twenty-four hours a day, anticipate his toilet needs, dress him in his favorite clothes, feed him from his favorite side, or switch on his favorite TV program.

Will he have trouble adjusting to his new routine? Sure he will, but not half as much trouble as you will have. You will be shocked by the apparent "I-don't-give-a-damn" attitudes of the aides until you realize that these people cannot afford the luxury of emotional involvement. You will be distressed when you see your child battling a juicy cold or scratching a mosquito bite, forgetting that he had colds and mosquito bites and upset stomachs and bumps and bruises at home. You will feel that he is not having sufficient contact with "normal" children until you remember how often the "normal" world has shunned him.

No, there is no "perfect place," but there are facilities which can treat with near perfection the particular condition of your child. This is why it is so vitally important that he be properly placed. In searching for a resident facility for your child, bear in mind that it should include the following features: (1) total rehabilitative services; (2) a policy whereby a certain time limit and specific goal is set for each child; (3) a location situated "where the action is" and not out in the boondocks; (4) a pleasant atmosphere with proper recreational and social opportunities for both sexes; (5) a total assurance in writing that you are not giving up your child to the will and whim of the institution.

If you've ever spent time in a hospital, you know how much visits mean. Unless your child is so retarded he doesn't recognize you, your visits will really be important to him. This is especially true if he is in a rehab center learning to walk, talk, and develop hand coordination. He'll want like crazy to show off what he's learned to the people he loves most. Make no mistake. The things he is learning do not come easy. He is working hard and needs your encouragement.

Don't expect miracles. Progress will be slow.

3

"Why Does It Take So Long?"

You're the parent of a CP child. You know the score, you know the statistics. A CP child is born every fifty-three minutes. There are more than 990,000 CP children and adults in the United States. You grit your teeth whenever an acquaintance arches an eyebrow and asks, "Was there anyone else in the family like HIM?" or "Is it safe for my Johnny to go near him?" for you know that cerebral palsy is neither hereditary nor contagious.

You also know that there are many types and subtypes of cerebral palsy, and such an endless combination of these types that no two CPs are affected in exactly the same way. The type and degree of disability is initially dictated by which combination of cells in what area of the brain are damaged.

You know all this—and more. Yet there is so much you don't know. And the frightening part of it is that the more you talk with doctors, the more you realize that they don't know either. The greatest "area of the unknown" shared by you and the professionals is in predicting how much progress your child will make—and how long it will take.

Still, the medical picture is not all that negative when compared to what was known when I was a child. Today, at least, doctors can recognize CP, and their guess as to which child will benefit from therapy and which child won't is a lot more educated.

But in the dark ages of the early 1930s too many doctors pretended to know more than they knew. Witness some of the things my parents were told about me, things I understood perfectly even though I was not yet able to talk:

"His brain is being crushed."

"All he needs is a few electric shock treatments applied to the soles of his feet."

"He'll outgrow it by his seventh birthday."

"Don't feed him. Don't bathe him. Put him in a dark room and forget about him." (Parents and professionals alike fail to realize that every child, whether he can speak or not, is fully aware of what is being said in front of him. I am still angered by those who insist on referring to me in the third person: "What does *he* want for dessert?")

Then there were the relatives and friends, always ready to volunteer a diagnosis, a course of action, or a remedy. The diagnoses, usually negative, were given to spur my parents into a course of action. The courses of action, also negative and summed up in the four words "put the boy away," were suggested by those who could think of no remedy for my condition. The remedies prescribed were, to say the least, pretty wild.

Perhaps the most bizarre cure came from an alleged Indian princess my mother met in the park. The princess believed that I couldn't walk or use my hands because my arms and legs were weak. She reasoned that man's strength comes from the earth, that worms are earth in living form, and that application of earthworms to my limbs would give me strength. Of course, the worms had be fried and mashed first . . . .

My mother tried it—once.

But let's return to the more pleasant present. Witchcraft is virtually gone from the medical scene. The old wives' tales have been told and almost forgotten. Rehabilitation is much more of a hit than a miss proposition. In short, real help for the CP child is at hand.

I've said before that the most effective therapy program is one where the child is getting daily treatment in a resident facility. This is without question the most desirable setup. Unfortunately, this type of facility is difficult to find. You are more likely to find that your child must attend an out-patient clinic or rehab center.

Wherever he goes, the success of his program and the rapidity of his progress will depend upon what he does, not in the therapy room, but in his own home. So often I have seen a child walk beautifully for his therapist and spend most of his home hours in a wheelchair because his parents do not encourage him to leave it.

This is the pitfall of being an out-patient: The real struggle to overcome one's disability takes place at home. If you think you had responsibilities before, what with feeding, dressing, and bathing your child, wait and see what's in store for you.

Fighting yourself will be the toughest part. Since your child was born, you have gotten into the habit of doing everything for him. Now, suddenly, your thinking has to be

13

reversed. You must allow him to spill food on your clean floor, walk without the security of your arms, and take himself to the bathroom. You'll worry a lot, but in the long run it will be worth the worry.

In all likelihood, your child will slowly learn to do things for himself—and do them slowly. His slowness will irritate you at times, but this irritation will be offset by your pride in his accomplishment.

On the other hand, you must not allow his slow pace to become his life style. Gently encourage him to quicken his pace, and to develop methods of cutting down the time it takes for him to be independent. You will have to be directly involved in pushing your child to move faster, because the rehabilitation centers are not likely to do so. All too often, a rehab center is a world unto itself, and a self-perpetuating world at that. It is a world where the child is told "Take it easy," "You still have twenty minutes to get to physio, so don't hurry." This gives the child the feeling that there is one set of rules for "normal" people and another set of rules for people like him. He sees his father do the Dagwood bit in the morning, but it doesn't register with him because he has never been told that this is going to be a part of his life someday.

I said before that the rehabilitation center is all too often a self-perpetuating organism. By this I mean that the longer your child takes to learn to do as much as for him as possible, the longer the professional staff can safely look ahead to secure jobs. This is why so many rehab centers have gone on from basic therapy to education, prevocational training, vocational training, and sheltered work-shops—but seldom job placement.

There are many practical shortcuts which your child can

14

take to speed up his activities of daily living. For example, if it takes him a long while to button his shirt, perhaps he could learn to put it on over his head partly buttoned. Loafer type shoes will eliminate tedious lacing. And the list goes on forever. Ask any occupational therapist.

There is considerable debate among professionals as to whether parents should have a picture in their minds of what their children will be like in ten years.

One view is that if the parents can visualize their child accomplishing a certain feat, they can project this confidence in him. From my own experience, I know that if I can picture myself doing something, I can usually learn to do it, so that the idea of planting a picture in a child's mind of what he will be able to do is not as farfetched as it may seem.

I'm afraid, however, that I am more inclined to agree with the opposing view. Many doctors warn that both overestimating and underestimating a child's capacity to achieve is extremely dangerous. If the parents underestimate their child, they may well hold him back from doing as much for himself as he can. If the parents overestimate the child's potential, they may cause him severe emotional difficulties by putting on pressures he cannot handle.

Speaking of parents, staff members of many rehab centers devote much time to getting parents to talk to each other, the theory being that the way one parent has solved a particular problem in caring for his CP child will be of value to other parents. This is undoubtedly true, and very often much is accomplished when parents compare notes. However, I should caution you not to be overwhelmed by the "older and wiser" parent who seems to have all the answers. This parent may indeed have "all the answers" for *his* child, but that doesn't mean he is right about *your* child.

One thing you the parent can be sure of, however: In ten years your child will be at least twice the size he is now, weigh at least four times what he weighs today, and be faced with problems far different from the simple feeding, dressing, washing problems he faces today.

One might almost say that the degree of physical progress your child makes in the next ten years is irrelevant. More pertinent is your own realistic awareness of your own limitations. Let's take a minute to list the things you won't be able to do in ten years for your child:

(1) You will no longer be able to lift and carry him about as you do now.

(2) For his mental health and proper development, you *should* no longer bathe or toilet him, especially where the child is of the opposite sex.

(3) You will not be able to make up his whole world, for he will need peer companionship of both sexes even more than he does now. (This is true regardless of the presence or absence of retardation.)

(4) Your physical strength, mental concentration, and emotional state will no longer enable you to give as much of yourself to your child.

Playwright Clifford Odets has said, "The job of a parent is to make himself unnecessary." This statement is no less true for the parent of a cerebral palsied child.

How can this be accomplished? This question will be discussed in the next three chapters.

4

Setting Priorities

Look at any fund-raising campaign poster of United Cerebral Palsy or some other agency designed to serve the multihandicapped. What do you see? You see a child either proudly taking his first step or sitting in a wheelchair with a look of deep sadness on his face, almost as if he were apologizing for not being able to walk. It is indeed unfortunate that *walking* seems to be so important to parents, doctors, and therapists. In my view, it is at the bottom of the rehabilitation priority list.

I consider walking unimportant for several reasons. First of all, among the cerebral palsied adults I have known, the most successful and socially accepted are those who live in wheelchairs. Any CP who is even moderately affected will never be able to walk without that weird scissor gait which causes him so often to be mistaken for a drunk. Secondly, the CP who walks lives on the edge of normalcy. Because he can walk, it is difficult for him to relate to his CP brothers who are in wheelchairs. And yet he can never quite walk well enough to be considered "normal" by the so-called normal world. This state of limbo is not easy to live in.

Thirdly, there is the matter of safety. A person whose walk is unsteady is far more likely to fall, be hit by a car, or be physically attacked by others than is a person in a wheelchair.

Lastly, it has been my experience that an intelligent CP in a wheelchair is more likely to get a chance to use that intelligence. I know of many CP college graduates who, because they can walk, have chosen the line of least resistance and are working as runners on Wall Street or allowing themselves to be exploited in sheltered workshops. A CP of equal intelligence, confined to a wheelchair, *must* find ways to use what he has learned because he has no alternatives.

Don't misunderstand me. There are advantages to walking. If I have overstated the disadvantages, it is only to equalize all of the pressure coming from the other direction.

Society demands certain things from everyone. The priorities you set for your child and those which he sets for himself (they will vary slightly) must be in harmony with what society demands, at least to the extent to which he will need to depend on society, and to the degree that he accepts the dictates of society without compromising his own principles or life style.

With this in mind, I have prepared a list of priorities which every CP should try to adopt as his own:

(1) He must have a deep and abiding faith in his own

being a full-blown person goes the responsibility of being a member of the family unit and later of the community. Unless this sense of responsibility is instilled, your child, carried away by his own power, could become a monster who literally plays the role of house dictator. A well-developed psyche can easily take a swat on the bottom.

There is in the psychology of behavior modification a technique known as intermittent reinforcement. This simply means that instead of rewarding your child every time he does something right, you reward him intermittently. When, for example, he feeds himself without spilling and you reward him by letting him stay up for his favorite TV show, the next time he feeds himself as well he is not rewarded. Perhaps two or three times later you may give the reward again in a similar way, and then perhaps six or seven times will go by before his efforts are recognized.

What does this mean? Well, psychologists have found that this form of intermittent reinforcement instills in the child an "I-won't-take-no-for-an-answer" attitude. While this attitude may not be vital for the so-called normal individual, it is essential to the survival of the handicapped person. Persistence is perhaps the greatest quality a handicapped individual has going for him

If you were to take the same child and reward him every time he did something that pleased you, he would grow to adulthood with the feeling that he must be immediately gratified for his efforts, and when he was not gratified, he would give up.

The child who possesses a strong sense of his own sexuality is least likely to have to prove it later on. Men and women secure in their own sex roles will enjoy life more fully and can cross over traditional lines of mental attitude and physical occupation without feeling threatened. It is the secure man who can openly cry when it is time for tears, or can happily do housework while his wife brings home the bacon. Conversely, a secure woman knows that there is more to life than being somebody's wife or mother. She is an interesting person in her own right and will not fall apart when the people who have depended on her no longer need her.

You may not think so now, but your child, regardless of his disability, will one day find himself in the above situations. And even if he doesn't, his *true* value of himself will enable him to cope with situations which might otherwise be intolerable.

The second priority, encouraging your child to do as much for himself as possible in whatever way he can, may turn out to be one of the most difficult tasks for you to live with. It is easy enough to say in the abstract, "I don't care how he does it as long as he does it." But what about the stares and scowls of those who will see your child feeding himself with his foot, typing a letter with a stick fastened to his forehead, or putting on his trousers with a hook-stick held in his teeth?

These for you are the difficult times. Unfortunately, you will not feel the elation most parents feel when their child learns something new. Intellectually you will be glad that he has learned or been taught a new accomplishment. But emotionally you will wonder whether this accomplishment will be appreciated by society and whether it is right for you to be proud.

At this point I think it is important for me to remind you that your role as a parent is indeed to make yourself unnecessary. The accomplishment is more important than the method your child uses to achieve it. Here the end does justify the means. If self-sufficiency is the goal, then the road to that goal must be a freeway in spirit.

You will notice that in the third priority I shifted for the first time from general philosophy to specific activity. It was not by chance that the first of these specifics listed was self-care in the bathroom. Recently, I was called in to counsel a twenty-six-year-old man who, along with his family, sought advice regarding his educational and vocational future. I found out that this young man, whom I will call Ben, had been attending a junior college, and that his mother made this possible by hiring a fellow student to feed, dress, and toilet him. Ben's mother freely admitted that if toileting were not involved she would have to take far less from her limited finances to pay for Ben's care, for toileting is obviously the least desirable type of personal assistance to have to perform. I know of several mothers who find it repugnant to toilet their own babies and push toilet training to the point where psychological problems crop up later. How can one expect a stranger to toilet an adult without some financial compensation?

Besides, if your child marries another handicapped person (and this will be discussed later) he will have to care for his own needs because the one he marries will not be able to help him. And if he doesn't marry, his parents are not going to be able to lift him onto the toilet or into the tub. If he is in an institution, he must wait patiently for an attendant to be available unless he can toilet himself. So you see, whichever way your child's life goes, independent toileting is a must.

For three of the reasons given above, priority 4, getting oneself dressed and in and out of bed, is essential: if he should marry another handicapped person who cannot lift him; if he remains at home and you are too old to lift him; or if he is in an institution and must wait for an attendant.

In this matter of dressing, the real secret to independence is intelligent choice of clothing. Generally, your child will find it easier to put on a pullover shirt than to try to fasten buttons. This means, of course, that trousers with zipper flies are better than ones with buttons. Unless there is a medically prescribed reason, your child should never wear laced shoes. There are enough varieties of loafers, moccasins, and other types of slip-on shoes available that there simply is no reason why he should be bothered with laces, even if his hand control is reasonably good. The same is basically true for girls' clothing, for with the advent of stretch fabrics, even no-fasten underwear is available. Clothing which must be fastened can be equipped with velcro.

As far as getting out of bed is concerned, I should recall here that while I was living with my parents my wheelchair was automatically put out of my reach when I went to bed. The reason is unimportant, but the result was that I was left stranded and could not have gotten out of bed in case of emergency. Also, if your child can transfer from wheelchair to bed and back, he can transfer from wheelchair to *anywhere*. This is particularly important in self-toileting, and for transferring in and out of cars. Remember that transportation may well be your child's greatest practical problem on the socioeconomic level, and if he must be lifted in and out of a car, it will not be easy for him to get a ride.

The fifth priority, personal hygiene, begins with an attitude. Your child must *want* to be clean before he begins to work at it. While instilling in a child a penchant for cleanliness can be overdone with drastic psychological results, a healthy desire to be socially acceptable is a plus in your child's personality. I know too many handicapped people who honestly feel that in the light of all their other disabling problems, personal hygiene is too picky a virtue to bother with. While this attitude can easily be understood, it is not to be tolerated by the thinking parent. Some CPs have perceptual problems which render them unable to know when they are clean and when they are not. In these situations outside help is definitely appropriate. Incidentally, awareness or nonawareness of personal cleanliness has nothing to do with intelligence. I know one young man who has been severely held back vocationally because he is not pleasant to be near. This person has a very high intelligence and could be successful in various fields of employment.

The sixth priority, dealing with communication, is one of the most difficult to achieve. The term "intelligible speech" is so ambiguous that it has no meaning. Speech which is intelligible to you and other members of your family may be totally unintelligible to outsiders. It may be difficult for you to believe, but many highly intelligent CPs have speech which is totally intelligible to *them,* and they cannot understand why words which sound so perfect to their ear are not understood by anyone else, even another CP.

There is a good chance, though, that if your child can make himself understood verbally by his family, not just you, others who become close to him will learn to understand him equally well and that this encouragement will do more to improve his verbal communication than all the speech therapy he may receive. Like any other therapy, such as physical and occupational, there is always the danger that what is learned in the therapy room will not carry over into the outside world.

But now let us assume that your child is incapable of speaking. There are alphabet boards, word boards, electric typewriters, and other devices now being developed which will enable him to communicate with other people.

In priority 6, I warned against a code between you and your child. The reason that any kind of code is dangerous to your child's future development is that as long as he is able to let you know, for example, that he is hungry by crossing his legs, he will not have the motivation to try to communicate more effectively with you or anyone else. CPs, like most people, will always choose the line of least resistance. Besides, how will the teacher or the neighbor down the street know that when your child crosses his legs it means that he is hungry? Even if I were to choose a less ridiculous code, such as smacking his lips, sticking out his tongue, or pointing vaguely in the direction of his mouth, there is every possibility that his gestures might be misunderstood.

There is a vast difference between the type of code I have just described and what is known as "nonverbal communication." Communication on the nonverbal level can be highly successful and in some ways more desirable than limited intelligible speech. Before your child has had schooling enough to use the devices described above, he must depend on the look in his eyes, the expression on his face to convey his feelings and needs. However, an even more important form of nonverbal communication is physical contact. As you hold your child in your arms, you know what he is trying to tell you, particularly on the emotional level. My chapter on touching will go into this aspect of human relationships more fully. Suffice it to say that even the child with perfect speech should not be deprived of the "stroking" experience of nonverbal communication.

Priorities 7 and 8—drinking through a straw without spillage and brushing his teeth—are self-evident, and, I believe, adequately explained, as are priorities 10 and 11—self-feeding and miscellaneous essential tasks. But priority 9, education and training for employment, deserves its own chapter because of its scope and life-long ramifications. There is, perhaps, no area more vital to the future of your child.

6

Learning, Working, and Living

The title of this chapter was not chosen lightly. Education, employment, and the enjoyment of life are separate entities, one of which may or may not lead to another. The question of education for the cerebral palsied child is so complex that a close examination of its theories, practice, and goals is mandatory.

As a parent, your attitude about education for your child is going to depend initially upon your evaluation of his mental and physical condition. If your child has been labeled "retarded" by the professionals, and you happen to concur with this label, you might well ask: "Why bother to educate him?" By the same token, if he is so physically involved that a true picture of his intellectual ability cannot be obtained, you may have similar doubts as to the value of education for your child.

The human mind is so complex that no one can really predict how much your child, retarded or not, is going to be

30

able to learn. I know a CP adult who is moderately retarded (approximately 65 IQ) who has attained a B.A. degree. Memory and intelligence appear to have little correlation, and much of what this man has learned was learned by rote. Yet because of his experience in college, he is a fuller and happier person than if he had just been written off as a retardate incapable of learning—particularly higher learning.

My own view of the severely disabled CP who is unable to communicate verbally with others, and therefore is an unknown quantity, is that the first thrust educationally should be in the area of reading. A severely disabled CP needs the fictional and nonfictional world of books to expand his own limited experience. A person who can read is never lonely, even if he is shut off from the world by institutional life or kept prisoner in his own home by architectural barriers of steps.

But let us assume that your child is not that severely disabled, that he may indeed be able to attend special classes or even regular classes in public school. Let us further assume that he is of normal or even above-normal intelligence. Do all these pluses add up to a reasonable guarantee of a good education?

Before we answer this question, let us go back to the homebound child. What kind of education will he get? If he is lucky, at least as lucky as I was, the board of education in his community will provide him with a home tutor. From my own experience I can tell you that this is both good and bad. I received, during my primary and secondary years of schooling, vital individual instruction and personal interest which I could never have received in a classroom. Because my classroom was my living room, my curriculum was not colored by the teacher's need to plan a viable program which would include the mentally retarded. I had the freedom to go as far as I wanted to in any subject without being held back by others who could not maintain my learning pace.

On the other hand, I was not stimulated by classroom competition or friendships made in school. Also, my teacher came to my home three times each week for an hour and a half per session. This meant that the bulk of what I would learn was dependent on my willingness to do homework and on how much of this homework I would allow my parents to do for me.

But now let's look at the CP child in public school. How much better off is he? In some states education for the handicapped is not even mandatory. When it is, there are states which will grant high school diplomas to students who have never learned to read or write. The rationale here is that a diploma will make it easier for the graduate to find employment. Is this true? For the illiterate graduate, and even for the one who has received quality education, the answer, sadly, is no.

A moderate disability and a good education are by no means a guarantee to a successful career.

Discrimination in employment is a fact of life with which your child, if deemed employable by training and placement personnel, must live. We have not yet reached the point in our society where, as the President's Committee on Employment of the Handicapped is wont to say: "Ability Counts!" Ability only counts when it suits the employer's public relations image to "hire the handicapped." If I seem to be overstating the situation, it is only because I feel compelled to balance out the picture of sweetness and light presented by the President's Committee and by other public and private agencies that work with the handicapped.

It is easy enough to prove that more handicapped people, especially the cerebral palsied, are relegated to sheltered workshops than are employed in competitive industry. The sad fact is that no sheltered workshop has as yet found a way to utilize the tremendous resources of the human mind. It is standard procedure to place a CP, regardless of his intelligence, on an assembly line where he must struggle to put to use that which he can often least control: his hands. I must also add here that all too often even the best workshops prefer to keep in sheltered employment those who could well advance into industry, for the simple reason that the workshop must maintain production in order to secure subcontract work. The rationale in all this is that the person who is being held back is "more comfortable" in a setting where he is physically superior to his coworkers, and that, as one who is less disabled than the others, he has the responsibility to keep the workshop going for them. Conduct a little research in your own area and see how many workshops for the handicapped employ job-placement personnel.

One more warning about workshops. It has been my experience that many of these are not content with exploiting the handicapped by holding them back. They must go one step further by charging the parents a fee for the privilege of having their child say, "I am going to work."

The fact is that sheltered workshops are not the answer for even the most profoundly mentally or physically handicapped person. It seems to me that a viable alternative would be for federal, state, and local governments, together with voluntary health agencies, to subsidize private industry to find an appropriate place where the individual could perform within his ability the task he is best suited for and enjoys the most. This should all be done with the understanding that every worker will receive the legal minimum wage. I believe that this plan, though seemingly costly, would result in the tax charge being transformed into a tax payer.

But what can you, the parent, do about the problem of work?

Today, when our nation's small businessmen are experiencing hard times, more and more parents are leading their handicapped children into self-employment. Most of these enterprises are doomed to fail, not only because of the times, but because the young businessman has had insufficient training in running a small business. The Small Business Administration has no special department for the handicapped. The Office of Vocational Rehabilitation will not train the budding small businessman, because, very often, he has been declared "unemployable." Where, then, is the CP businessman going to pick up the know-how to run his own business?

Chances are he won't. Junior's business will probably become a family project. Dad will decide what type of business is "best for Junior" and will take care of the purchasing, bookkeeping, and tax accounting. Mom will line up the customers to buy Junior's indispensable product, whether they want it or not. Sister will keep the establishment clean and wait on trade because Junior doesn't have the hand control to make change, and Brother will get Junior to the store on time and set him up in a good spot in the store where all Mom's friends will see him, but where he isn't in the way.

Seriously, the CP who actually researches and opens his own business, perhaps with a little physical and financial help from his family, stands a far better chance of making it.

Here I must go back to my own story. From the time I was six or seven years old, my parents instilled in me the fact that my mind was all I had. They probed with me the possibilities for future careers which might be within the realm of my own interests and personality. By the time I was thirteen, I had already done a juvenile form of individual counseling, and had begun to develop my writing talent. At the age of twenty-two I had my own newspaper column, and nine years later I began practicing my skill as a counselor professionally. All this without a college degree. I cannot help but wonder how far I would have gone careerwise if those early seeds of direction had not been planted by my parents.

The ironic part of all this is that my parents never honestly believed that I would ever work. Why, then, all this preparation? The reason my parents instilled in me an appreciation and respect for my own mentality is that they wanted me to enjoy life. Also my parents wanted to make sure that if I thought in terms of work at all it would be in the area of creative professions rather than industry. I know of too many CPs who have been brainwashed by parents and professionals alike into thinking of themselves as potential white-collar or blue-collar workers rather than people with professional or paraprofessional careers.

But let's get back to my parents' primary purpose in making me aware of my mind: the enjoyment of life. It was they who first introduced me to the philosophy that the highest achievement a person can reach is a thorough appreciation of the joys of living, and that while it is perfectly true that work can be part of that appreciation and is often necessary for survival, it is not an end unto itself. We work to live, we do not live to work. America is only now beginning to realize the fallacy of the work ethic, and to see that automation requires that we find happy and personally meaningful uses for leisure time for all, including the handicapped, especially those individuals who are so severely disabled that they cannot possibly work.

But—leisure time can only be meaningful when there is a choice between it and work. Proof that the federal government in fact does not expect the handicapped to work in gainful employment is that more money is allocated for recreation for the handicapped than for all other rehabilitation services put together, including medical services, education, vocational training, and job placement. This allocation, earmarked for recreation, obviously does nothing to help the CP adult achieve independence or an awareness of his intrinsic value as an individual. It merely lulls him into thinking that society expects nothing more of him than to go to summer camp, swim, bowl, and make (not create) unidentifiable artsy-craftsy objects which will never be marketable or add in any way to his support.

So far as the handicapped are concerned, there is an important difference between living in time and living in space. Time is the period we spend between doing something and doing something else. Space is the period between nothing and nothing. Good conversation, verbal or nonverbal communication with friends, reading, really *looking* at television, creative activities such as painting, singing or playing music, writing, cooking and sewing, going to good parties (rather than dull ones) all fall into the category of "doing something." In addition, falling in and out of love, feeling strongly about a cause, or sharing a "golden moment" (which may be happy or tragic) with someone you really care about are also "doing something." However, the cerebral palsied cannot participate in any of these nonwork activities unless they know who they are and have a healthy respect for their own mentality—whether or not they happen to be classified as mentally retarded. Among the most self-contented people I know are those who register a low IQ. This is especially true if they are not pushed beyond their abilities, while at the same time not allowed to think of themselves as "retards."

Your cerebral palsied child will have a much happier life if he realizes that his main reason for being born is to enjoy every moment and every facet of living.

7

The Untouched

Actress Jane Pickens, a regular on cerebral palsy tele-
thons, relates the story of her visit to a private rest home
where her CP daughter has lived for some years. During
this particular visit, Miss Pickens noticed a severely disabled girl sitting by herself near a window. The actress
cheerfully went up to the girl, said a few words of greeting,
and warmly put her hand on the girl's shoulder. At the
touch of Miss Pickens' hand, the girl burst into uncon-
trolled tears. Afraid that she had done something wrong,
Miss Pickens ran to an attendant and related the incident.
The attendant looked at the visitor and said, "Miss Pickens,
don't you realize that this is probably the first time anyone
outside this home has touched that girl?"

While this story was used for dramatic effect on the
telethon, it is nonetheless an accurate reflection of the
experiences shared by most profoundly and moderately
disabled CPs. The CP is the "untouchable" of the twentieth

century. I know of no other disability which carries with it more tragic lack of physical contact with other people—even other CPs.

The truth is that our society is revolted by the cerebral palsied, and the cerebral palsied, like any other group of people, reflecting the attitudes of society, are compelled to reject themselves and each other.

What causes this mass revulsion? Look at any TV commercial or movie. Almost invariably, the hero or heroine is physically perfect and cosmetically attractive. Thus, by the time a person of the Western world is four or five years old, he is already conditioned to admire and want to be with the best-looking physical specimen he can find.

Our Judeo-Christian world is hypocritical as compared with more "primitive" societies. In these societies a deformed or sick baby is left on the hillside for nature to take its course. Being civilized, we make sure that no such barbarian practice befalls our children. We see that they get the best medical care in order that they may grow to adulthood—an adulthood of loneliness, prejudice, paternalism, neglect, and rejection. I'm not saying that the primitives are right in their very direct approach to solving the problems of the handicapped, but I am suggesting that if we are going to save the life of a handicapped child we as a society are responsible for the happiness of that life. A few years ago, in an article called "Would You Make a Pass at a Girl in a Wheelchair?," I pointed out that a person in a wheelchair is seldom if ever regarded as a love object, and certainly not as a sex object.

But let us return to that teen-age girl who was so tenderly touched by Jane Pickens. Unless this girl was an orphan, it is pretty safe to assume that her parents found it more convenient to "put her away" in a home. Unless the decision to place her was based on the factors mentioned in Chapter 2, it would appear that rejection of this child came rather early in the game. Any touching that was done by the parents was probably coincidental to physically caring for her. I would suspect that she was seldom cuddled for cuddling's sake.

Human beings need physical contact with one another at all times, but there are two periods in life when touching is most important: the first in early childhood, the second during adolescence. There is general agreement among pediatricians and child psychologists that the first four years are the most formative in a person's life. Eric Berne and Thomas Harris in their books on transactional analysis refer to the pleasant experiences during this period as "stroking." The term is quite appropriate because paramount among these "childhood recordings" are the fondling and cuddling the child receives. The more frequent the stroking, the greater is the child's feeling of external approval and self-acceptance. Conversely, lack of stroking is likely to give the child a generally negative attitude about himself and the world around him. Naturally, most of this stroking is given or withheld by the parents, although others may be involved.

Most of the stroking given very young children takes place during feeding. For the cerebral palsied child, this is a particularly good time for stroking. First, it is a solid block of time which the parent *must* set aside several times a day. Second, along with the beneficial stroking goes another feature essential to the child's survival: feeding.

Generally speaking, the cerebral palsied child must be fed with more care and skill than other children. Because of excess motion, drooling, or choking, only half of what the child is fed is actually digested. It is not uncommon to see an older cerebral palsied child or adult who is undersized and underweight. This is directly due to poor nutrition in the early stages of life. Also, the athetoid burns up more energy in three hours than the "normal active child" does in a whole day.

An even more serious point: Careless or hurried feeding, where the CP child's head is not supported, can send food into the lungs, causing pneumonia and possibly death. Your reassuring touch can help relieve the muscle tensions which may cause your CP child to choke.

The establishment of priority 1—a feeling of self-worth and acceptance of one's own sexuality—is mainly dependent upon stroking.

Assuming that the teen-age CP has known physical affection as a young child and that the idea that he is a sexual being has already been implanted, it is during the turbulent time of adolescence that this self-image is put to a test. I feel that I was luckier than most teen-age CPs of today because I was spared the rigid regulations imposed on the adolescent by many rehabilitation centers and special schools. Somehow, these places of learning and training manage to keep the sexes apart while making the individual feel sexless. This would appear to be a contradiction, since one would assume that a young man would feel masculine in company with other males and that a young lady would feel very feminine among other females. I have observed that such is not the case, for the simple reason that no person can be fully aware of his own sexuality unless he is aware of the opposite sex.

The happiest times of my teen years were spent on the

41

streets of New York City where I was free to try to impress girls I liked. True, most of my attempts met with failure, but I had just enough successes to make me reasonably sure that one day I would marry and share real love. Girls did kiss me and tell me how handsome I looked. They sat on my lap and put their arms around me. In other words, I was stroked. Also, there were occasions when girls who were distressed by personal problems actually found comfort in my arms, even if those arms were not as gentle as I wished them to be. As I look back on these experiences, platonic as they were, I realize that without them I might have questioned my own sexuality and never established a lasting relationship with any woman.

I will have more to say about touching in my chapter on marriage and parenthood.

This time of adolescence is so complex for the CP. It is the time when he must somehow make sufficient peace with his own disability that he can make the transition from childhood to adulthood as smoothly as possible. It is the time when the teen-ager must look in the mirror and, because he is a teen-ager, be dissatisfied with what he sees and somehow figure out a way either to change what he sees or accept it. This is also the time when he can never be quite sure how seriously other people take what he is saying, or trying to say. Indeed, it is a time when he must prove to the world that he exists.

The nonhandicapped adolescent can prove his existence, or attempt to, by rebelling against authority. The handicapped teen-ager finds this much more difficult, because he is dependent upon the authority against which he most needs to rebel: namely you. The handicapped teen-ager usually has no peer group with which to align himself.

Others in his situation are no better off than he and thus can give him no comfort. Commiseration is for the elderly, not the teen-ager.

So he must go it alone, trying to make sense of himself and the world around him.

What can you do? Nothing. The man-to-man talks of the Andy Hardy era are no more—if they ever were real. It is during the teen years especially that your child wants a parents, not a pal. If you tried to be a pal, you would be invading his privacy. The only thing you can do is goad your child into rebellion, take your lumps, and be glad that he has the spirit to fight. He will need that spirit all of his days.

It is almost as important for your child to witness touching as to experience it. Seeing his parents display open affection for one another is reassuring, especially if he is likely to hear occasional harsh words between his parents. Remember that your child is more dependent on you than most "normal" children. "What will happen to me if Mommy and Daddy go away?" is at the top of your child's "fear" list.

Before I close this chapter on touching, I should mention a couple of other areas which are vitally important to your child's growth. If he has a problem communicating verbally, owing either to severe speech defects or to difficulty mastering language (such as that of the aphasic child), touching may offer him a means of communication more effective and self-rewarding than any gadget educators or scientists might dream up.

Adolescents who have no physical disability at all live in a period when half-formed ideas cannot adequately be expressed in words. This is also a time when adults seem to misunderstand every word the teen-ager says. The term "sensitivity training" has been expanded and distorted to the point of nonmeaning. Yet the technique whereby people communicate their nonverbal feelings has been extremely helpful to teen-agers. Unfortunately, professionals have not used it with the handicapped to any real extent.

Do the professionals also consider the cerebral palsied as "untouchable?"

The final aspect of touching I'd like to mention in this chapter concerns the opportunities your child must be given to handle everyday objects. Developing what doctors call kinetic sense is an important part of learning. After all, one day your child is going to have to be able to distinguish between a nickel and a quarter simply by sense of touch. Also, the more objects your child becomes familiar with, the fewer things he will be afraid of and the more things he will learn to avoid because they are dangerous.

8

"You Want to Get—What?"

Yes, that's right, the time has finally come. He says he wants to get married. You never really believed the day would come. It's one thing to take care of a CP child because he's yours. But who in her right mind, a perfect stranger, would want to take on that kind of responsibility?

Well, the fact is that your child, who is now old enough to run his own life, has found someone to marry, someone who loves him as much as you do but does not want to be his parent, someone who is going to depend on him as much as he depended on you all these years.

And even as you realize this, the question arises within you: "Why does he need to get married? He's free to come and go as he likes. He's respected as an adult and doesn't have to prove anything. Why is he asking for trouble?"

He is not "asking for trouble." Rather, he is asserting his right as an adult to what boils down to a "license to touch." We have already discussed the importance of touching in the life of the young child and the teenager, but the need to be stroked does not magically end with adolescence. The need for physical affection is lifelong, and whether society is ready to recognize it or not, marriage among the handicapped is much more than platonic. I have too often heard, "Isn't it nice that John and Mary are getting married. They need the companionship."

Sure, handicapped people get married to avoid loneliness—who doesn't? But never underestimate the sexual needs or the need for simple cuddling which is the primary motivating force in any marriage.

I wish I could say that whether your child marries or not is strictly his own business and none of yours. Unfortunately, this is not true unless he is physically and economically independent. If your child is to marry and you are involved in any way in the practical problems of living that this marriage will create, you have a right to be consulted.

Just as it is unfair for you to impose your fears and prejudices upon your child in attempting to prevent his marriage, it is equally unfair for your child to find his adult happiness within the protection of your continued care.

I know a CP couple who brag about their happy marriage and two beautiful children. True, their marriage is very happy and their children are very beautiful, but the catch is that the husband's mother cares for the children and the wife's father supports the little family.

There is really nothing wrong with this setup—until something happens to grandma and grandpa. Any marriage that depends on *specific* individuals for survival is in danger and is also grossly unfair to the individuals upon whom it depends.

If you will recall my chapter on priorities, I put at the

top of the list your child's awareness of himself as a person and as a sexual being. Inherent in this priority is your obligation to develop in your child the conviction that one day he *will* marry. However, this conviction must be modified to say, "One day you will marry, if you prepare yourself for marriage—a marriage which does not include us, your parents."

Just as you have an obligation to make your child believe in himself and in his ability to love and be loved, so does he have an obligation to prepare himself for the responsibility which goes with that privilege. If he is going to fit you into his marriage plans, you have every right to say, "No!"

How can you tell in advance whether your child can find marital bliss on his own? His dating habits are a good tip-off. Does he rely on you for transportation? Has he dated a number of girls on his own, or has he relied on you to "fix him up"? Does he pay for his own dates? Is he working?

Of course, if your CP child is a girl, the same questions should be asked about her fiancé. In addition, remember that it is important for her to feel secure in her sex role as well. Throughout her time with you, she must be allowed to play housewife: learn to cook, sew, do other household chores, and above all, to love.

Why is the subject of sex education, dating, and marriage for the handicapped child such a fearsome area for parents? From the many fathers and mothers I have counseled through the years comes my observation that at the root of their fears is the awesome possibility that one day there will be *two* handicapped people in the family: their own child and the one he marries. If parents had any assurance that their handicapped child was capable of attracting and marrying a "normal" person, they would not look upon the entire subject of heterosexual relationships with so much trepidation.

Statistics do show that the handicapped are inclined to marry one another. But if the tests of real independence described above prove positive, the family is not gaining another cripple; it is rather allowing two handicapped people to live together legally and care for each other, with one ability augmenting the other. The example most convenient for me to use on this score is my own marriage. When Joy and I married she was more mobile than she is now, but basically we helped each other in the same ways we do today. She feeds me, buttons my shirt, shaves me, and transports me in our car. Since she is a dwarf just over three feet tall, I, in turn, open and close doors and windows, boost her up onto "big people" chairs, get for her things which are beyond her reach, and perform those everyday activities which require strength.

All this is wonderful and inspiring, but remember that in early stages, when your child is first thinking of dating and eventual marriage, he is not thinking in terms of another handicapped person. After all, your child is a reflection of society, and society considers the handicapped untouchable. So, given a free choice, your child would prefer romantic involvement with a "normal" person.

This does not happen very often, but when it does, the parents of the handicapped child are usually less concerned. If you become such a parent, you may well be fooling yourself, because the opposition your child will meet from potential in-laws is more heartbreaking and harder to live with than the mere physical solving of problems involved in marriage with a handicapped person.

48

I realize that at this point it takes more than a bit of imagination for you to picture your child as a parent. No one needs to tell you the responsibilities involved. Even though scientific research is beginning to suspect that a degree of heredity does exist with cerebral palsy, it is still more likely that if your CP child marries another CP their children will be perfectly normal. I know of no instance where heredity has been a factor in the birth of a CP child.

I indicated above that it is totally unfair for your CP child to expect you to take care of any grandchildren which may result from your child's marriage. Without getting into any religious issues, my consistent advice to CP couples who wish to marry, but know that they cannot take care of a child, is sterilization. I usually recommend a vasectomy because this surgical procedure for the male is so much simpler than sterilization for the female.

Even though we are not on the subject in this chapter, I should like to add that if your child, male or female, is so severely disabled that institutional life is inevitable, sterilization is essential. I have seen too many state institutions for the retarded (a category which usually includes the nonverbal CP of normal intelligence) where female inmates are victimized—primarily by attendants, not male inmates —and babies often result. For example, in one "school" in New York state, two hundred babies are born each year to female inmates. The reason it is important to sterilize your institutionalized son is so that he cannot possibly be blamed for any of these tragedies.

However, in spite of my strong position on the need for sterilization of the institutionalized, I am vehemently opposed on civil rights grounds to compulsory sterilization laws passed by the state. These laws dehumanize the handicapped and take out of your hands and your child's a decision which is of a most personal nature and must not go outside the family.

But now let's bring your child back out into the world and return to the subject of grandchildren. Even if sterilization is against your religious convictions, please consider the ethical question: Is it moral to deny your child the right to marry based on a practical situation which is beyond his control? In other words, if your child and the handicapped person he marries are able to carry on the business of marriage without too much help from other people, and only the presence of a child would create real tensions, why shouldn't this couple be permitted and encouraged to avoid this problem?

My point is that your CP child's marriage, if approached realistically by the parties concerned, will have no more and no fewer difficulties than your own marriage. It may work; it may not work. If it does, it will be because two people met, fell in love, became each other's very best friends, and have achieved as close to total communication as is possible between two people. If their marriage does not work, it is highly unlikely that it will be because of the physical handicap.

In this chapter, and every one of those which preceded it, I have tried to get across one point: The cerebral palsied child, while as unique in detail as any other child, faces now, and will face in the future, his version of the challenges presented by life which everyone faces. If you keep this basic concept in the front of your mind and heart, you will one day know the pride that every parent feels for the adult who was once your child.

9

You and Your Life

In this book we have been concerned with your child and have done considerable projecting into the future regarding him and his life.

But what of you and your life? Just how much are you expected to sacrifice in order to bring about the development of an independent adult from what is now your helpless child? I've observed that most parents of CP children give too much of themselves—not too little. This is why, when the "child" is of adult age, so many parents are reluctant to let go and allow him to live his own life. The parent has invested so much in this child that the feeling of being indispensable has become not only comfortable but necessary for survival.

I cannot overstate the importance of *you* maintaining *your own* identity and your own outside interests. Above all, you must believe in your own mortality. I have said this before, but it is worth repeating: You are not going to outlive your child. He will either marry, as described in the previous chapter, live on his own, or reside in an institution.

Do not count on relatives to take over where you leave off.

How is it possible for you to "do your own thing" without neglecting your child or involving his brothers, sisters, aunts, or uncles? Fortunately, an increasing number of high schools are training students in what they must know to be a skillful babysitter for a child who might have an epileptic seizure (as many CP children do), throw himself out of bed through involuntary motion, wet the bed (even in his teen years), or have little or no speech. If you want to have the freedom to which you as a person are entitled, try to encourage a high school in your area to put this training in as part of its curriculum, if it isn't already there. Another procedure which will set you free is for you and parents of other CP children to operate a babysitting pool where one parent will sit for your child while you go out, and you will reciprocate in kind.

Vacations are always a problem for a family with a handicapped child, but this problem is not insoluble. Camping out, if you bring along the proper equipment, will not only be a joy for you, it will be a necessary training experience for your child.

While I have said that relatives should not be imposed upon, it is equally true that there is no reason in the world why grandma can't take your handicapped child while you go on vacation if she is also taking any of your other children. The handicapped child should not be a burden, but neither should he be left out of the family unit.

There is one activity connected with your child which is vital to his future and yet can provide you with an outside interest. I am speaking of political action. One tremendous failure I have found common among parents of CPs is their seeming inability to join together politically to lobby on the local or national level for or against legislation which directly affects the cerebral palsied. Many good bills, such as that which would grant tax relief to working handicapped adults, never got through Congress because parents did not express themselves on this issue. On the other hand, a bad bill which requires that all developmental disability programs serve primarily the mentally retarded passed because parents of the mentally normal CP children did not speak up.

The most active parent group is that which represents the mentally retarded. The blind and their parents are also active in lobbying for legislation, as are the parents of epileptics.

You may say that you would not know where to begin because your child has all of the above disabilities along with his cerebral palsy. There may be some validity in this feeling, but the fact remains that the parents of CPs are conspicuous by their absence in any expression of political action, be it demonstration or letter writing. These activities will not only help your child and others, they will open for you new areas of interest which might go well beyond the concern you have for your CP child.

I know that it has been hard for you throughout this small book to imagine the future. The present is so difficult to live with. But if you are able to look ahead at all, the writing of this book has been worthwhile.